Also by Robert Magarian

My Father, The Doctor

A Memoir

Robert Magarian

Dedication

To My Father, Leon Der Magarian, MD.
You taught me why we are on this earth.
You are loved, and are always with me.

৯০•৫৪

To all Armenian families whose ancestors
were murdered in the Hamidian Massacre in 1894-1896,
and the April 24, 1915 & 1923 Genocide

"And God shall wipe away every tear from their eyes. There will be no more death, nor sorrow, nor crying, neither shall there be any more pain; for the former things have passed away. Behold, I make all things new"

Rev. 21:4-5

Acknowledgments

Writing is a lonely task, which I fully enjoy because it puts me in another world. Having a team that helps bring life to my work is exciting. Among those deserving special acknowledgment are:

My life's partner, Charmaine, for reading the manuscript and providing helpful comments.

Many thanks to the following readers for their comments, corrections, and great insight into this work:

My cousin, H. Gary Apoian (author/attorney).

My nephews, Kevin and Timmy Magarian.

Thanks to my niece, Sarah Lodes, for her investigative work.

In remembrance of my teacher, Carolyn Wall, author/teacher. You taught me so much, and I'm forever grateful, dear lady. So sorry you had to leave us this year. You are sorely missed by so many writers.

Best Cover Designer: Peter O'Connor in the UK. He

designed the covers for most of my books. He can be reached at www.bespokebookcovers.com

Best Print Formatting and Publication Person: Amy Atwell, Author E.M.S. Amy is a jewel to work with and very efficient.

My family for their love and support. Love you all.

Introduction

This is a story about Dr. Leon Magarian, who lived tragedy and triumph. Born in 1882 in Armenia, a nation proud of its history and the first nation to adopt Christianity as it's national religion in 301 AD. He grew up in western Armenia under domination of the Ottoman Empire, and in the latter part of the century, his Christian family, endured intense, unavoidable hardships, injustices, and cruel blows of Turkish cruelty.

To escape the increasing hostilities toward the Armenians, Leon and his family journeyed to America in 1912 to East St. Louis, Illinois. His older brother Armanag and his wife Gulvart had a son, Alphonse one year later. Three years after his birth, the family faced further tragedy. Alphonse was kidnapped and brutally murdered.

Leon pursued a career in medicine and set up practice in East St. Louis as a physician and surgeon in 1921. The doctors at that time only had x-ray, blood work, and urine analysis—no CT scan, MRI, or PET scans. There was far less technology with greater reliance on doctor-patience relationship. Doctors worked long hours and made house calls. His son Bob learned from his dad a couple of practices in medicine that must be followed in making an accurate diagnosis: (1) listen to the patient, and (2) show compassion for them.

The turning point in the history of medicine came after the '50s. During that period, physicians had the autonomy to deliver highly personal health care, because federally mandated regulations were few and constraints from insurance companies were almost nonexistent, and the doctors had the authority to deliver highly personal health care in private practice.

Modern medicine differs drastically from the '50s, shifting from a paternalistic house-call model to a highly technological specialized and data-driven industry. Today's practice of medicine is a focus on chronic diseases, personalized medicine, surgical complex procedures and greater understanding of genetic and complex conditions.

Part One

Armenia: The Homeland

CHAPTER
1

My father, Levon Der Philibosian was born in the ancient land of Armenia in 1882, known in biblical times for its sacred Mt. Ararat, Noah's Ark, and the Garden of Eden.

Gregory the illuminator brought Christianity belief to the Armenians, who are proud to be the first nation in the world to adopt Christianity as its national religion in 301 AD through the efforts of King Tiridates III. The first church in the world was built in Armenia. Mt. Ararat, Armenia's national symbol, is a source of cultural and historical pride where Noah landed his ark after the waters of the World Flood subsided. Armenians saw themselves as the people of the ark.

"And the ark in the seventh month, on the seventeenth day of the month, came to rest on the mountains of Ararat" (Genesis 8:4).

As an ancient people, Armenians are proud of their rich biblical history and culture, where existed the Garden of Eden and Noah's Ark landing upon Armenia's sacred Mt. Ararat, which are mentioned in several passages: Jeremiah 51:27, Ezekiel 27:14, and 38.6. Jeremiah mentions three provinces of Armenia: Ararat, Minni, and Ashchenaz. Ezekiel mentions Togarmah, which is thought to be Armenia, and Isaiah 37:38 mentions Ararat, which was the central district around Mount Ararat. In Jewish usage, Ashkenaz is equated with Armenia. In Armenian literature, the Armenians are called "the Ashkenazi nation."

The Armenian language is unique in that its alphabet was invented around 405 AD by Mesrop Mashtots, making the Armenian alphabet one of the most ancient alphabets in the world. The world's first textbook of arithmetic problems was created by an Armenian mathematician.

In the nineteenth century, Armenia was a nation on the eastern edge of the Ottoman Empire (also called the *Turkish Empire*).

The Armenians called their homeland *Western Armenia* located between the Black and Caspian Seas, the Caucasus Mountains and the Mediterranean Sea.

The Ottoman empire began to fracture long before the empire collapsed entirely. Independent movements began to flourish. Several Ottoman territories became independent including Turkish nationalism, Arab nationalism, and Armenian nationalism were among the most prominent.

The Ottoman Empire was in a dire financial crisis. All legal authority became concentrated in the hands of the sultans. Resistance arose, particularly among a group of dissidents known as the Young Turks.

In this century, the Armenians were a developing Christian nation with many notable intellectuals, which did not set well with their neighboring, Islamic imperialistic Turkish Empire.

Trouble was brewing on the horizon.

Part Two

Hamidian Massacre

CHAPTER

2

The First Genocide of the Armenians occurred during Sultan Abdul Hamid II's reign of the Ottoman Empire, who developed a hate for the Armenian Christians and considered them a threat to the Empire's Islamic character. Consequently, he initiated and orchestrated the sacrifice of 350,000 Armenians from 1894 to1896, known as the Hamidian Massacre. In addition, thousands suffered unspeakable hardships in their native villages in Western Armenia, causing them to seek refuge in the Eastern part of their country. Local Kurdish Tribes and other Muslim villagers were encouraged to participate in the killing and looting of Armenians.

The Second Genocide of the Armenians occurred on 24 April 1915, the Ottoman authorities arrested and deported hundreds of Armenian intellectuals and leaders from Constantinople, which became the capital of the Ottoman Empire in 1453, and whose population grew to 700,000 in the 16th century. With the founding of the Republic of Turkey in 1923 the name changed to Istanbul in 1930. At the order of Talaat Pasha, 1.2 million Armenians were sent on death marches into the Syrian desert. The deportees were deprived of food, water, and subjected to robbery, rape, and finally slaughtered in the Syrian desert. The survivors were dispersed into concentration camps. In 1916, another wave of massacres was ordered, leaving about 200,000 deportees alive at year's end. In December 1920, the Soviet Union and Turkey invaded and throttled the two-year-old Republic of Armenia. Three separate Russian Red armies under Lenin's orders swooped down from the north. Simultaneously, the Turks under Mustafa (Ataturk) Kernal, in callous violation of the armistice of World War I, invaded from the west and southwest. Defenseless in the face of the overpowering military aggression, abandoned by the isolationist Allies, the Armenian Republic lost its independence, its culture—it's all.

(Notice: Some facts above were taken from "The Cross and the Crescent," by Lindy V. Avakian, page 102, USC Press, publisher).

At present, Mount Ararat is no longer considered in Armenia because the country was overrun by the Young Turks in 1921, and it is now considered to be in the territory of Turkey.

Part Three

A Bullet for Talaat Pasha

CHAPTER

3

(This chapter is paraphrased by the author, taken from "The Cross and the Crescent," by Lindy V. Avakian, Chapter Twelve, pp126-132, USC Press, publisher.).

Talaat Pasha, "The Monster," (a name given to him by the surviving Armenians whom he tried to exterminate) was facing his last days as his executioner, Soghomon Tehlirian, swore in his youth that he would find the man responsible for the destruction of his home and the deaths of nearly two million of his countrymen. Soghomon took up position outside unit number 4, on Hardenbergstrasse street, located in the Charlottenburg-Wilmersdorf district of Berlin, Germany on March 15, 1921. At 10 a.m. a puggy Turk, who Soghomon felt had to be Talaat, but needed proof before the kill, emerged from his front door this cloudy morning, glancing cautiously in both directions while Soghomon lurked in the shadows of an alley. The overweight Turk started walking in a thoughtful and focused way as if he had the desire to accomplish something. Soghomon was in pursuit staying a safe distance behind him. When the Turk reached number 47, he entered the unit known to be occupied by Turkish devils in hiding. At eleven o'clock, the obese Turk left and returned to his own home.

Was he really Talaat?

One of Soghomon's co-horts, Hazor, learned from an Armenian officer in the Berlin police, that he would allow Hazor and Soghomon to examine the alien visa files. As they examined the photographs, they saw the man they were following and felt he was Talaat. In the process of viewing the photographs, an overseas cablegram from Federation Headquarters in Boston arrived. Soghomon's face turned white as he read it.

Hazor wanted to know what it said. "They've learned the name of the heavy Turk we've been following. "Who is he?" Hazor asked.

"Talaat!"

In examining the original photo, they realized Talaat had his face altered surgically. After three years of giving his life in search for Talaat, Soghomon's constant surveillance of the Turk had revealed that Talaat seldom deviated from his daily routine. He usually left his house around 10 a.m. and returned at 11. That time schedule would cost him his life. The plan was to execute Talaat between 10 and 11 a.m. The morning of March 15, 1921 was overcast with snow falling, which turned into a drizzling rain. When Talaat came out of his house, Soghomon Tehlirian rushed to stalk the former Prime Minister of Turkey, the first modern architect of the crime of genocide, following him from twenty feet behind. The street was almost deserted, except for a few stragglers whose heads were hidden beneath their black umbrellas. Being within firing range, Soghomon kept his finger tightly on the trigger of his Mauser. He quickly crossed the street and doubled back. Now, Talaat approached coming a few yards between them. Soghomon raised his Mauser automatic and pointed the muzzle at Talaat's head. His eyes widened in fear. His mouth opens as in protest. He glanced around looking to turn. Fear of death filled his pudgy face. Soghomon fired once, standing with the smoking gun in hand. No need for a second round. Talaat collapsed, his body sprawled at the curb, his face half submerged in a puddle of water. The human who walked the earth on all fours was dead.

Part Four

Philibosian Family

CHAPTER

4

In the 1800s in Armenia, young men who aspired to become priests would typically seek training and ordination within the Armenian Apostolic Church. This involved a structured process including education and progressing through minor orders, ultimately leading to the major orders of presbyter (priests).

My grandfather, Sarkis Philibosian, was born in 1846 in the village of Keghi, a district in the province of Erzurum located in Western Armenia under the Ottoman Empire. Keghi is known for its mountainous geography and a large prosperous Armenian population that was wiped out during the Armenian genocide. It was home to a sophisticated culture with many village churches, and a strong focus on education, despite the threat and conflict with Kurdish and Turkish neighbors. The primary occupation for Armenians in Keghi was agriculture but commerce and crafts gained importance. Keghi was home to many prosperous Armenian merchants who grew wealthy through trade.

The name Sarkis means "rainbow." In his early teens he probably attended the Monastery of Saint Minas of Kes near the village of Kes for his education and the priesthood. Sarkis likely received religious instruction and theological education within the monastic or church settings. The specific curriculum and requirements would have varied depending on the specific region or monastery. Before becoming a priest, young men would typically be ordained into the minor orders, which were preparatory stages. These included becoming an Acolyte (Pokhasats), Sub-Diaconate and Diaconate. After progressing through the minor orders, young men would then be ordained into the major orders, which included the presbyterate (priesthood).

The Armenian Apostolic Church has a history spanning over 1700 years, dating back to the first century when it's believed to have been founded by Apostles Bartholomew (Nathanael) and Thaddeus, while Armenia officially adopted Christianity as its state religion in 301 AD. The church's roots are traced back to the Apostolic age with St. Gregory the Illuminator playing a crucial role in establishing the church in the 4th Century. He was a key figure in the early spread of Christianity, particularly in Armenia. Born in Cappadocia, he later became the first Catholicos (Patriarch) of the Armenian Apostolic Church. He is revered as a saint for his role in converting Armenia to Christianity and is considered the patron saint of the Armenian Apostolic Church.

The Cathedral of Holy Etchmiadzin is in Vagharshapat, Armenia, a significant church in the country, was built on a spot where St. Gregory had a vision of Christ. The cathedral dates to the 4th Century, and is reckoned the oldest Christian cathedral in the world.

At his ordination my grandfather chose the name "Magar." Reverend Sarkis (Magar) Philibosian (b.1846) met and married Hachatoun (gift of the cross) Mary Demerjian, my grandmother, who was born in 1853 in

Karboz village in the province of Erzurum, which in the 1800s was in Western Armenia (controlled by the Ottoman Empire) was a significant village with a mixture of Armenian and Turkish populations. It was a relatively large community with its own social structure, traditions, and economic activities. The village played a role in the broader economic and social landscape of the region, engaging in agriculture and animal husbandry.

My grandparents married in 1870 (she was 17 and he was 24) and they established a small church in Keghi. In addition to attending to his flock, my grandfather would visit other villages to hold services.

Mary and Sarkis had four children – Armanag (b. 1880, name means "Armenian"), my father Levon (b. 1882, name means "lion" signifying strength and courage), a daughter, Maria (b. 1884)) and Kordan (b. 1886, name means "guidance" or "leader").

Armanag Der Philibosian, the oldest sibling, quit school after the eighth grade. He married Gulvart R. Ovian (b. 1886) and their first child, Aznive was born in 1899, and their second child Roxie, in1901 followed by Helen in 1904 who died at birth, Vivien, in 1905, also died at birth. Armanag had a penchant for business, and everything he attempted succeeded. He looked to the future harboring a great desire to go to America to build a business and to avoid the threats of the Turkish Sultans.

Levon Der Philibosian went to college in Constantinople where he earned a BA degree in theology and mastering French. He spoke French fluently and developed a strong liking for the French people.

Maria Der Philibosian, my aunt, married a man whose surname was Mooshegian. They had one son, Arsen, who emigrated to the U. S. in 1912 and settled in Detroit, Michigan. Little else is known about my aunt other than she died a natural death around 1915.

Sultan Abdul Hamid II, who hated Armenian Christians orchestrated the sacrifice of 350,000 Armenians from 1894 to1896 (Hamidian Massacre).

The Philibosian family escaped the Hamidian Massacre, and after the turn of the century, the family realized their safety had worsened and knew their future emigration to America had arrived. Many Armenian men were traveling back and forth between the U.S. and Armenia to gain work.

In 1907, my uncle Armanag and my father Levon decided to go to America to establish a residence for the family. The journey was a significant undertaking facilitated by the prearranged emigration agency to travel to the Northern France City of Le Havre ('the harbor"), a major port city (Port of Le Havre) situated on the right bank of the estuary of the river Seine. They boarded the French ship La Provence, and arrived in New York, New York on 28 December 1907 after a seven-day journey. Armanag had purchased second class tickets on the ship which was a level under the ship's first class.

Armanag was 27 and Levon 25. At Ellis Island, the brothers had to register a family history and my uncle registered the family name as Magarian and not Philibosian. He took his father's ordination name "Magar" and added "ian" to it. His reasoning was: Americans would remember it better than Philibosian. My father allowed it, but I don't believe he agreed with my uncle. My reasoning for the change is that my uncle thought with a business mind and failed to honor my grandfather, Reverend Sarkis (Magar) Philibosian's surname. (*My uncle's action has always bothered me, even though I was born Magarian.*)

Most of the Armenians at that time were in transit for manufacturing towns like New York City, Providence, RI, East St. Louis/Granite City, Illinois, and Detroit, Michigan, or settling in rich farmland like California's San Joaquin valley. These immigrants were mostly men, many of whom went back and forth between North America and their homeland several times.

The Philibosian (now Magarian) brothers traveled by train from New York to East St. Louis, Illinois with the great Mississippi river separating it from St Louis, Missouri where many Armenian families settled. They settled in what was considered at that time, the southern part of East St. Louis where several factories employed hundreds of immigrants from several nations. Armanag saw this as fertile ground for building a business. He opened a bakery in front of their home at 19 N. 16th street. My father, Levon worked the bakery, which he didn't enjoy. As a man with a bachelor's degree, who loved the French language, and an avid reader, had it in his heart to become a college professor one day.

Uncle Armanag became known as AD (Armanag Der) Magarian, a wealthy baker with the nickname, "King of Little Armenia." He even did banking for the Armenian families. After three years of missing the family and being unhappy in the bakery, with no future in sight, Levon, now Americanized to Leon, told his brother he was going back home. AD agreed that Leon should go back and bring the whole family to East St. Louis because many reports from the newly arrivals told them about the Turks creating much more havoc among their people. AD's plan was to remain behind and continue to expand their business in the area.

In 1910 my uncle, Kordan Der Philibosian, entered Yeprad College, also known as Euphrates College, which was a significant educational institution primarily serving the Armenian community in the region of Harput (now part of Elazig, Turkey), during the late Ottoman Empire. It was founded in 1878 by the American Board of Commissioners for Foreign Missions and evolved from a theological seminary established in 1852.

Yeprad expanded into a college in 1878, and eventually became Euphrates College after being initially named "Armenia College." It focused on educating clergyman for the Armenian Evangelical Church and later expanded to provide general education in English. Armenian influence played a crucial role in cultivating the Armenian language and culture in the college, including the publication of a newspaper called "Yeprad" in Armenian and printing religious and school books in Armenian script.

In 1912, my father, Leon, after being back from America for two years, realized it was now time for the family to go to America. He wrote his brother, Kordan, demanding that he leave college immediately and come home because the Turks' animosity towards the Armenians was intensifying, and the family were preparing to leave for America.

Kordan wrote to his oldest brother, Armanag, demanding that he tell Levon to stop pestering him to come home that he had no intention of leaving Armenia. Due to his stubbornness, he stayed back as the family left for America. Some months later, the family got word that Kordan's college was severely impacted with several faculty members arrested, tortured, and executed. Kordan

Der Philibosian, my uncle, along with all the other Armenian students were taken from the college and lined up against the building and shot. Then the college buildings were occupied by the Ottoman military and used as a training camp and hospital. Euphrates College was officially closed after the Republic of Turkey was founded in 1923, and nothing remains of its buildings today. Like many Armenian villages in Western Armenia, my ancestors' hometown, Keghi, and its population were displaced or killed during the Armenian Genocide of 1915.

Part Five

Bound for America

CHAPTER

5

In spring of 1912, my father, Leon Der Magarian, took charge of preparing the way for the family's trip to America through the same emigration agency used in 1907. The family members who joined my father on the journey were: Armanag's wife, Gulvart (26 years old), her daughters: Aznive (13 years old) and Roxie (11 years old); and Leon's mother Mary Demerjian Der Philibosian (59 years old). Her husband, Father Sarkis Philibosian died of pneumonia.

Their journey was the same as taken in 1907 by Armanag and Leon where they traveled to Western Europe and boarded several train changes through France of which one brought them to the City of Le Havre and the Port of Le Havre. Hundreds of Armenian families were waiting in the port town to board the ships to America. Leon being fluent in French took it upon himself to interpret instructions from French into Armenian so his countrymen could board the ships.

The Philibosian family boarded a French ship to America and arrived in New York Ellis Island seven days later in May of 1912. They traveled by train to East St. Louis, Illinois and set up housekeeping at the Bakery/house residence on 19 N. 16th street. On September 3, 1913 a boy was born to AD and Gulvart Magarian, who they named Alphonse.

Next to the bakery/residence was a saloon over which was a brothel operated by a husband-and-wife team, Charles and Garnet Droit. AD pushed to shut down the house of ill repute known as The Droit Resort.

After several complaints logged by AD Magarian, the police arrested the couple. Soon after, Magarian's 3 year old son, Alphonse, was kidnapped.

⅓•⅔

As reported in *The St. Louis Star and Times*, St. Louis, Missouri, Friday October 6, 1916, page 10:

"While two searching parties today were looking for Alphonse Magarian, 3 years old son of the "King of Little Armenia" who disappeared from his home (19 North Sixteenth Street) in East St. Louis, Tuesday night, the father, A.D. Magarian, a wealthy baker, offered a reward of $2000 for the child's return.

A bloodhound was used in an unsuccessful attempt to find the boy yesterday.

The dog took the scent from some of the child's clothing and from a go-cart and ran to sixteenth street and Broadway, a block away, where he sat down and howled. Twice the bloodhound repeated the performance but went no further than a block from the home. The police interpreted this as indicating the child had been taken away in an automobile.

A child in the neighborhood said he saw the Magarian boy in the alley Tuesday afternoon and a strange man nearby. The search for the missing lad continued today, the father heading one party and the mother another. Mrs.

Magarian hasn't sleep since her son disappeared.

The police believe Magarian may have unwittingly offended some of his countrymen and his son was kidnapped for revenge. Magarian is well to do, but no demand has been made on him for money."

℘•℘

[Taken from McLaughin, Malcolm, *Power, Community, and Racial Killing in East St. Louis*. New York: Palgrave Macmillan, 2005.]

Well-to-do Armenian baker, A.D. Magarian, the "King of Little Armenia" in East St. Louis, pushed to shut down a house of ill repute over a saloon next door to his bakery/residence. The "Droit resort" as it was referred to by one paper, was a brothel operated by husband & wife team, Charles & Garnet Droit.

After Magarian lodged several complaints, police raided the brothel on September 30, 1913. Garnet Droit was held on the charge of white slavery in conjunction with operating a "disorderly house." She & the girls were held on bond. After their release, the Droits and several coconspirators plotted their revenge.

On October 4, Alphonse Magarian, the 3-year old son of A.D. Magarian, was kidnapped, murdered and beheaded in retaliation. To cover their tracks, the gangsters framed the murder on a prostitute at the brothel, then placed her murdered body on the railroad tracks to make it look like suicide.

Alphonse's headless body was discovered in a rubbish dump, or "ash pit" as they were sometimes called, one block from the Magarian home, ten days after he disappeared. The body was wrapped in newspaper.

His head was found in a gunny sack at another dump a week later. The police initially suspected Turks -natural rivals of Armenians then.

Lex Droit & Charles Bergholz of East St. Louis and two others were tried by jury and acquitted of murder in connection with the boy's death. Droit and Bergholz were convicted & sentenced to 15 years in the Southern penitentiary for the crime of kidnapping however.

Sylvia Upton, a 16-year-old "inmate of the Droit resort" testified at all three trials that she overheard threats against Magarian after the police raid.

At the time of the trials, James Campbell was serving a 20 year sentence for robbery that would not expire until 1934, and was never tried on the kidnapping indictment. A fourth suspect, Danny Sullivan, was never apprehended.

ஐ•ରଃ

The loss of Alphonse became an incredibly difficult journey for Gulvart Magarian to overcome. She survived the tragedy by navigating through her grief by honoring Alphonse's memory, and with the strong support of her daughters Aznive (17 years old) and Roxie (15 years old), and concentrating on raising her one-year-old son, Albert Ararat Magarian, born in 1915. Gulvart had two more children, Anahid Octavian Magarian (b. 1917) and Alphonse B (Bus) Magarian (b. 1919).

The bakery business had expanded with the girls working full time, supervised by their father, AD. The girls complained to him that their uncle Leon wasn't helping in the bakery, but would only sit in a corner reading books.

That's when AD said that Leon, who had a prior degree and was more interested in academia than helping in the business, should go to school.

Part Six

Leon Prepares for Medical School

6

One evening their family doctor, Dr. Little, came into the bakery for some goodies and AD took the opportunity to tell him about his brother and asked if he had any advice for them about Leon's future.

Dr. Little asked Leon what his interests were. He said he loved French, but never thought about what he might do with it. He never mentioned his degree in theology.

After learning that Leon had a bachelor's degree, Dr Little said, "I'd recommend that he consider medicine. We are short of doctors."

AD asked how could they begin. Dr. Little recommended that Leon write Valparaiso University to inquire about their premed program, and with his credentials they could determine what courses he needed to complete. Dr Little had attended Valparaíso University's premed program, which was connected to Loyola University Medical School in Chicago where Dr. Little received his MD degree. He said he would be glad to write a letter of recommendation to both Valparaiso University and Loyola School of Medicine.

My dad was able to obtain a letter from his college in Armenia that confirmed his bachelor's degree in theology and a major in French along with his degree certificate. Leon wrote to Loyola University Medical School and provided them with all the information they requested. He learned that they required certain undergraduate courses he did not have before he could be admitted, and hence directed him to take the required courses at Valparaiso University in Valparaiso, Indiana, which wasn't far from East St. Louis.

Leon learned from reading their literature that there was an historical connection between The Loyola University School of Medicine in Chicago and Valparaiso University. The Chicago College of Medicine and Surgery was initially founded as the College Eclectic

Medical College in 1901 and became a medical department of Valparaiso University in 1902. The institution was finally purchased by Loyola University in 1917.

After two years of premed courses at Valparaiso from 1913-1915. Leon was admitted into the fall semester at Loyola School of Medicine in 1915. He graduated in 1919 with his MD degree and interned at Oak Park Hospital in Chicago from 1919-1920 after which he returned to East St. Louis to set up practice as a physician and surgeon. He received his registration certificate from the *State Of Illinois* as a *PHYSICIAN AND SURGEON* dated August 1921.

With financial help from his brother AD, Leon built a beautiful brick single story office building with three front windows one each side of the three step entrance with a canopy at 1511 E. Broadway that he moved into in early 1922.

On the center front window on the left side was painted my father's name and underneath was his title: "Physician & Surgeon." The other two windows as well as the three on the opposite side had metal designs embedded in the glass. The front yard of the building had a small grass area on each side of the sidewalk, which was enclosed by a metal fence and gate.

Inside, the office building had a beautiful terrazzo flooring that extended into both sides of two large waiting areas, and down a hall that ended into to a large room at the back used as a kitchen. Down the hall, on each side, were three examining rooms. Four- feet from the entrance stood a white three-foot drinking fountain.

Chairs lined up along the walls on both sides of the waiting areas with the secretary's desk against the wall in the left waiting area. Along the walls were pictures of medical scenes.

Adjacent to the building on the west side was Knewitz's Drug store and across the street in the middle of the block was Daut's drug store and on the same side, but down on the corner at 15th and Broadway was an Armenian family grocery store, Golden Rule. Continuing west on Broadway about a block away was Prompt Cleaners owned by the Marifian family, and across the street was Broadway Cleaners owned by the Chuchian family.

There were homes on the other side of my father's medical building, which extended east for one block. The inhabitants were a mixture of immigrants that had come to work in the factories that were a few miles south of the area. On the corner of 16th and Broadway was a grocery and butcher shop owned by the Ovian family. For many blocks on Broadway lived many Armenian families. Most of whom were close friends.

Earlier in 1920, AD Magarian had built a new two-story brick home in the northern part of East St. Louis at 1307 N 25th street, which was ten miles from their place of business, located in a beautiful developing area across from a magnificent park, *Jones Park*.

Part Seven

Romance

CHAPTER

7

In 1923, Dr. Leon Magarian had built a large practice and was on the staff at St. Mary's Hospital. In late September 1923, one of his patients, Pauline Struel, an eighteen-year-old, had come to his office with her mother complaining of something in her eye. Dr. Magarian found himself attracted to this young lady. During her second visit he became even more attracted to her and took her mother aside and asked if he could have her permission to take her daughter out for an evening meal. Hesitant, she told the doctor that she would have to discuss it with her husband and her daughter. She didn't know if Pauline would even be interested. After all he was some years older than she.

He looked over her records and found her address, which was only a few miles from his office, and that she worked as a telephone switch-board operator.

A week later, in the late afternoon, when he had finished seeing all his patients, and not having any house calls, Dr. Magarian slipped into his new Ford Model T and went to the Struel's house on Missouri Avenue just three miles from his office. He pulled into their driveway and stopped close to the front. He stepped out of the car and walked up the three steps to the porch and knocked on the door. He noticed a swing to his right that was attached to the ceiling with hooks and chains.

A tall man with thin light-auburn hair and stocky built opened the door, his expression serious, and not smiling. Leon introduced himself as Dr. Magarian and wondered if he could come in and talk with them. He learned that the man's name was Oscar and assumed he was Pauline's father. He was led into the kitchen where Pauline and her mother were seated at the round table having dessert and coffee. He saw Pauline sitting next to her mother in front of the refrigerator across from her father, who pointed to an empty chair for the doctor to sit.

"Would you like to join us for any dessert" Pauline asked. "We have cherry and apple pie and chocolate cake."

"Coffee would be fine," Magarian said.

The mother whose name was also Pauline got up and handed him a cup filled with coffee on a saucer. "Coffee milk is on the table," she said.

Leon nodded as he kept his eyes on their pretty daughter who looked down at her piece of pie at times in shyness.

"You are Armenian, correct, doctor?" Oscar asked.

"Yes, sir," he said, adding milk to his coffee.

"We're Germans," he said.

Leon nodded. Pauline looked up and smiled at him, but her mother was stone- faced.

"What brings you here, doctor?" Oscar asked.

Magarian had a hunch the father knew but he played along, hesitating for a few minutes. "I came to ask your permission to take your daughter to dinner, if she's willing to go with me. I find her to be very pleasant and would like to get to know her."

Oscar looked at his wife and then at his daughter.

"That would be up to Pauline, Oscar said, gazing at his daughter. Her mother just nodded.

There was silence.

They may not like her going out with a foreigner, Magarian thought. *I never had trouble interacting with Americans in Chicago.*

Finally, Pauline looked at her dad and mother and said, "I wouldn't mind if you both approved."

Oscar took his time answering. "I think that would be permissible, doctor."

Magarian was very pleased and finished his coffee and stood up "I must be going," he said.

Pauline rose and said, smiling, "I'll show you to the door."

When they stopped at the door, Magarian, being only five-foot-two, turned and looked up at the five-foot-eight lady and asked if tomorrow night would be okay for a casual evening with a meal at a little Armenian restaurant.

"I've never had Armenian food. I'd like that," she said as she opened the door. He stepped out on the porch and said, "Can I pick you up at seven?"

"Yes."

As he walked to his car, Leon felt a warm feeling come over him.

8

The next day, being Saturday, Dr. Magarian finished seeing his patients around 4:30 p.m. He had one house call to make and after that he drove to his brother's new home on north 25th street where he was living. In the home of AD and Gulvart Magarian included their oldest daughter, Aznive Apoian, her husband Henry Apoian, and their one-year-old son, Haig. The other Magarian children were Albert Ararat Magarian, Anahid Octavian Magarian, and Alphonse (Bus) Magarian, and Roxie Magarian who later moved to Los Angeles and married George Ovian.

The Magarian family now called Leon Magarian, "doctor," since he had finished his medical education, and established his practice in East St. Louis. He didn't think it was necessary, but was okay with it.

The doctor had told the family about his date this evening with an American girl, Pauline Struel. The family pressured the doctor to bring Pauline to the house after their dinner. Once his older brother AD nodded, he agreed.

It was 6:30 p.m. when my father arrived at Pauline's home. He pulled into their driveway and ambled out of his brand new Ford Model T.

The Model T was introduced in 1908, featuring a revolutionary design for its time, making it affordable and accessible to a wider audience. Key features included a light-weight, strong vanadium steel chassis, a simple and efficient four-cylinder engine, a planetary engine, a planetary transmission controlled by foot pedals, and a left-side steering wheel. Th engine produced 20 horsepower and allowed for a top speed of 40-45 mph. It was designed to run on gasoline, kerosene, or ethanol. The fuel tank was located under the driver's seat or on the back, and fuel was gravity-fed to the carburetor. The car had to be cranked in the front to *start it. Dr. Magarian purchased it for $269 in early 1923.*

Dr. Magarian ambled up the steps to the lighted porch of the Struel's home and knocked. The days were becoming shorter and the evening was pleasant. Pauline immediately opened the door, smiled and stepped out into the Autumn air wearing a light-blue, ready-to-wear house dress instead of an evening dinner dress, that hung loosely and down to the top of her ankles, that exposed black shoes with a leather strap. Since they were only having a casual dinner there was no need to dress up. She wasn't wearing any jacket since the weather was still very pleasant and she carried a small black cloth purse. He reached for her arm and guided her down the steps to his car, and opened the passenger side door and assisted her into his little car. After closing her door, he went around to the driver's side and reached in for the hand crank, which he inserted into a socket at the front of the engine. He made a series of ratcheting turns, to rotate the engine's internal parts, which generated the spark needed to ignite the fuel to start the car. He came back to the driver's side, replaced the hand crank and slid in behind the wheel.

"Your car looks brand new," she said.

"I just bought it a few months ago."

As he backed out of the drive, he told her he was taking her to an Armenian restaurant on Broadway a couple blocks from his office, and hoped that was okay. "The place is not fancy, but the food is excellent."

"That'll be fine," she said, smiling.

Once he came to 15th street, he drove south three blocks to Broadway, and then turned right and pulled up to the curb a few doors down from the corner and parked in front of Manoogian's Armenian restaurant. The front of the eatery had a large window that exposed a bright room filled with many tables covered in white linen. The sign above the entrance had the name: *Manoogian's Armenian Restaurant.*

The Manoogian's had been the doctor's patients since he opened his practice and he often enjoyed eating there.

He hurried around the back of the car to open Pauline's door and helped her out. They walked to the entrance and inside most of the tables were occupied with Armenian families eating and talking in Armenian. A few of the children were running around the room. A middle-aged, slender woman probably in her early sixties, wearing a white apron over a flowered house dress was in the back of the room talking to a thin, bald man about six inches taller than she. When he pointed to the front, she turned and immediately hurried to greet them.

"Doctor Magarian, welcome," she said gripping his hand and bowing. Then they spoke in Armenian. The doctor smiled. The lady turned to Pauline and said, "Please to have you at our restaurant. My name is Roza."

"I'm Pauline. Pleased to meet you, Roza."

"So pleased to meet you, Pauline. This is my husband, George." He was the man she was talking to when they entered. He nodded and moved to Dr. Magarian and said, "Doctor. Please, come this way." He led them to a smaller room off the main dining area into a room with four tables dressed very neatly in white linen and table settings. George held out the chair for Pauline and she sat. Roza brought them a typed menu. Most items were in Armenian with English translation under each item.

"What do you recommend, doctor?" Pauline asked.

He frowned and said, "You can call me, Leon."

Pauline shook her head no. "I couldn't do that." She quickly said, "What do you recommend? I don't understand any of this," she said, holding the typed menu. "It's all Greek to me." And smiled.

He laughed. "Not Greek. Armenian."

She smiled, again.

He liked Pauline's sense of humor.

"I think we should choose the family meal," he said, looking at the menu. "It has a little of each of our best Armenian dishes."

"I'd like that. I enjoy cooking and may even ask Roza how she prepares some of them."

He smiled. He was becoming more relaxed, and enjoyed being with her.

CHAPTER

9

Leon smiled to himself, somewhat surprised how Pauline enjoyed many of the Armenian dishes and how Roza took time to sit at the table with her and discuss some of the dishes. Roza gave her an extra copy of a typed book on Armenian cooking. He was very pleased the way Roza took to Pauline.

During the meal, Leon talked about his family and how they escaped the Turkish 1894 genocide in Armenia, and about the loss of his brother Kordan, and his father, a priest, who died of pneumonia, and how his brother AD established the bakery when they came to America.

While eating, he wondered how she might respond if he asked her on this first date to meet his brother and family. He would emphasize that they were very interested in meeting her.

Would she think I'm being too aggressive? he thought.

When they were nearly finished eating he asked her. To his surprise, she thought it would be nice to meet his family. On the way to his brother's home, he tried to put Pauline at ease with small talk about who she would be meeting, and how nice they were. Pauline became interested in his elderly mother, the only family member who couldn't speak English, and who was married to an Armenian priest.

Pauline told her date that she was Roman Catholic. He pulled the Model T up in the Magarian's driveway and helped her walk down the small incline to the sidewalk that led up to the house. They could hear family members talking behind the screened-in porch. When they entered through the screen door, three women met them at the entrance — Gulvart, AD's wife, their oldest daughter, Aznive, and second daughter Roxie. They greeted Pauline with open arms, smiling and saying how glad they were she came to visit them.

The doctor could see the smile on Pauline's face as the three ladies embraced her, who then led them into the living room where they saw AD. Albert, and Alphonse, whom immediately stood up when the couple entered. Leon introduced Pauline to them.

Pauline noticed the little elderly lady in a rocking chair behind AD. She was rotating beads on a rosary with the fingers of her right hand and moving her lips. Pauline went around AD to grandma Magarian, gripped her left hand into hers, and gave her a big smile. Grandma looked up and smiled back at her, not saying a word since she couldn't speak English.

"Hello," Pauline said. "I'm pleased to meet you."

Grandma looked up at AD and said something in Armenian, He relayed the message to Pauline: "She said, who is this lovely person." He then said something to grandma Magarian in Armenian, but never told Pauline what he had said.

Aznive told the doctor and Pauline that she and Roxie were going to help their mother in the kitchen and to prepare the dining area for some coffee and dessert.

AD led the couple into the large dining area directly

behind him and he pointed for Pauline to sit to his right as he sat at the head of the long table with his back to the windows. The other family members joined them. Pauline noticed grandma was left in her chair and she got up and went to help grandma to the table. All eyes were on Pauline.

Aznive and Roxie brought in platters of Losenogs. Gata, and Baclava and placed them in the center of the table. Soon Gulvart came in with an urn of coffee and set it on the dining room buffet.

The ladies poured the coffee for everyone and then sat. AD began passing the platters around the table starting with Pauline. "Please help yourself."

"It all smells so good," she said. "I've had Baclava, but not these others." She removed the pastries from the platters as they were passed to her and then cut them into halves and placed some on the doctor's plate.

All eyes were on Pauline. This is all very good, but I think I like the gata best because of its buttery flavor.

"Doctor told us you like to cook," Aznive said.

She looked at him. "Yes, I kinda compete with my mother who is an excellent cook. I'd like to try my hand at some of the Armenian dishes. Tonight, I was fortunate to get an Armenian cookbook from Roza Manoogian. She was so nice explaining the best way to cook some of the items by following her cookbook." The ladies looked at each other.

After everyone had finished eating, AD suggested they go into the living room. As they rose from their places, Pauline said to Leon, "I think I'd like to go. I need to prepare for church in the morning."

He nodded and they thanked everyone and walked to the door where Aznive met them with a covered plate and handed it to Pauline.

"Here's some of the dessert items that you might like to share with your mother and father."

Pauline thanked her and they hugged.

In the car, Pauline told the doctor that she really liked his family, especially Aznive, and that she had concerns since she wasn't Armenian.

He smiled. "That doesn't matter."

Earlier the next morning, Pauline had set the table in the kitchen, and was cooking eggs and pancakes, and had coffee ready for her father who liked it first thing in the morning. The Armenian pastry was kept warm in the oven. Oscar came into the kitchen as she just finished, and poured himself a cup of coffee.

"Did you have a good time last night with the doctor?" he asked.

"Yes," she said as she placed the eggs and pancakes on the table. "I met his family."

She saw the raised brow on his face. She moved the bread and butterdish in front of him, "They were very nice and I brought home some of the delicious

Armenian pastry, which I know you'll love."

At that very moment, her mother entered and said, "What smells so good? I don't recognize that smell."

"That's Armenian pastry," Oscar said. "She brought it from visiting his family last night."

"Oh-h-h-h, I see," her mother said. "Meeting his family after the first date." It was more sarcasm than a statement.

"Yes, that's what I was thinking," Oscar said.

"Don't read too much into it. It was nothing more than an evening of meeting other people. They all were so very kind and nice," she said as she placed the Armenian pastry in front of them.

"We're just asking, dear. No need to get huffy," her mother said.

"I know what you both are driving at. I do like the doctor, if that's what you are concerned about."

Neither parent said a word.

"What else is there to do around here?" Pauline said. "I really enjoyed myself. We never have anyone over and we never go to visit anyone. I'm lucky to have my girlfriend, Mable."

She stormed out of the room saying, "I have to get ready for church."

That afternoon the doctor came by to see if she'd like to go for a ride. The weather was nice and the sun was bright this Sunday afternoon in late September. She was pleased he showed up.

They continued dating for months. Christmas had come and gone. In early Spring the doctor noticed that Pauline's parents still weren't too friendly towards him, and he wondered if they didn't like him because he was Armenian and older than their daughter. During one of their dates, he asked Pauline about it. She told him she didn't want to bring it up just yet, but since he asked, she told him they were only concerned about receiving her help to pay off their house mortgage.

"I had to quit school after the eighth grade to go to work to help them."

"You mean they made you drop out of school to help with their bills?"

"Yes, it's common here in the U.S. for children, especially the girls, to quit school after the eighth grade and go to work to help their families."

He shook his head. "I'm sorry to hear that. Never would have happened in Armenia."

During the summer of 1924, the doctor took Pauline out for what he called a special dinner date. After finishing their meal, he reached for the small box next to his plate that Pauline had been eying all evening, and removed from it a small velvet box, He rose and moved to the chair next to her and removed the lid. He reached in and withdrew a gorgeous ring with many diamonds in a set etched in black. He took her ring hand and slipped it on her finger, and asked her to marry him.

Pauline admired the ring on her finger. "It's beautiful," she said with tears in her eyes. "I would be happy to be your wife. I love you and your family, but…" She stopped for a second, and then went on to say, "It's customary for you to ask my parents for their blessings."

"Why the sad look. Do you think they'll disapprove?"

"No, it's…" She stopped, again, and then said, "It has to do with their mortgage situation that I told you about."

He thought for a moment and said, "I want to meet with them."

"You do?" "What about?"

"Just set a time."

When Pauline got home that evening, she went into the living room where her father was sitting in his easy chair next to the radio, listening to Jack Benny and her mother was knitting a sweater in her rocker.

"I have something to tell both of you, she said, followed with a big smile.

Both parents stopped and looked up. Pauline knew what they were about to say by looking into their cool expressions.

She held out her hand. "I became engaged this evening to the doctor. He asked me to marry him and I accepted."

There were no congratulations, not even a 'We are happy for you, dear.' Just silence for a few moments.

"Well, what do you think?" Pauline asked.

"We know you're happy," Oscar said, "but you know our agreement,"

"What was that?" Pauline asked, knowing what was coming, but wanted to hear it from him.

Her mother answered instead, "The mortgage. It must be paid off before we can give our blessings."

Pauline darted out of the room and hurried up to her room.

A week later, the doctor and Pauline had planned a special dinner meeting with her parents, because Dr. Magarian said he wanted to meet with them. He wouldn't tell her why, but she felt like she knew.

Pauline had prepared the evening meal, and she and the doctor sat together across from her parents. After finishing their meal and dessert, Doctor Magarian turned to her parents and said, "Mr. and Mrs. Struel. I thank you for the kindness you have shown me these many months. You know by now that I am deeply in love with your daughter, and want her for my wife. I am told you won't give your blessing to Pauline to marry me because of your house mortgage. Is that correct?"

They sat in silence.

Oscar spoke, "We want what's best for our daughter and we think you would make her a fine husband, but we had this agreement between us for some time that the mortgage had to be paid off first before we could give her our blessing in marriage."

"Would you be willing to give her your blessings if I paid off your mortgage?"

Pauline's eyes widen as large as half-dollars. He hadn't told her.

Both of Pauline's parents looked at each other. He could see the surprise in their faces.

"You would do that for us, doctor?" Oscar asked.

"No. I would do that for your daughter."

Oscar said as he looked at his wife, "I believe I speak for both of us. We'd gladly give our blessings on the marriage of our daughter to you."

Pauline rose and embraced the doctor as he stood to shake her father's hand.

"Then we have an agreement?"

"Yes, sir," her father said, as he stood. "We certainly do"

Mrs. Struel standing, embraced the doctor, which greatly surprised him.

11

A month after the dinner with her parents, the doctor and Pauline were out this October Sunday afternoon driving east on State Street, a major thoroughfare that horizontally bisected East St. Louis into north and south areas. He came upon 25th Street and turned left heading north to a stop at St. Clair Avenue. He proceeded through the intersection, and drove over two parallel padded railroad tracks, arriving at one end of a beautiful park, Jones Park, on their right, and across the street on their left were several baseball diamonds. A half-mile down the road, was a fork in the road. The road to the left took them to his brother AD's home a block away, but the doctor chose the road to the right, which curved around the left side of the expansive park.

"I see AD's house over there," Pauline said, pointing to their left. "Will we be going there?"

"We will but first, I have a surprise for you and want to show you a little more of this area. I know we were here before, but there is more to see."

"What? A surprise. Give me a hint."

"You'll have to wait and see." He continued along the curve that went around Jones Park on Caseyville Avenue.

"Look to your right at the beautiful lagoon in the park. It has a pavilion where music is played on Sundays and there are canoes and rowboats to rent."

"It is beautiful," she said.

At the end of the curve there was a large fenced-in outdoor swimming pool in the park. He turned into the street that went around the pool and fifty yards from it was a baseball diamond to their right, surrounded by a large picnic area with a snack bar. The park covered many acres with trees and beautiful plants and flowers. He came back out of the park onto 25th street again and turned to his right heading back towards AD's home.

"Now the surprise," he said taking the road to the right again around the curve but slowed a block away at a road to his left that ran perpendicular off Caseyville Avenue, and pulled up into a dirt drive next to a new brick home that was still under construction and needed landscaping.

"How do you like it?" he asked.

"Very nice."

"This is going to be your new home. I'm building it for you. I have the plans that I want to show you when we get to AD's. I know it's not finished, but from what you see, how do you like it?"

Pauline's right hand went to her mouth. She was speechless. "I can't believe this. You really mean this is going to be our home?"

"Of course. Where did you think we were going to live?"

"I never gave it much thought." She leaned over and hugged him. "Thank you so much. I never dreamed I'd have a home like this. And a beautiful park across the street."

He hesitated for a second. "Now we need to set a date

for our wedding. The builder told me the house would be completed by November 1st. "Have you given that any thought?"

"Of course.

Still sitting in the Ford Model T, they thought about a couple dates close to the time when the house would be finished. After some discussion they set the date for Tuesday, November 4, 1924.

As it turned out, November 4th was a big day for the couple. Besides their wedding day there was a lot of activity in the national election for president.

The couple had planned their church wedding and reception at St. Henry's Catholic Church located at East Broadway and North Sixth Street. While the doctor wasn't catholic he honored his future wife's wishers to be married there.

There was a problem, however. The church wouldn't allow the couple be married in the church. They had to have their ceremony in the priest's parlor because Dr. Magarian was married and divorced back in Armenia, and his ex-wife was still alive living in Michigan. A divorced man couldn't be married in a Catholic Church unless his prior marriage had been legally declared null and void by the church through an annulment, or his former spouse had died. Divorce does not end a marriage in the eyes of the church. The doctor wasn't in agreement and thought the rule illogical, but didn't object to please his bride.

Part Eight

Marriage

12

The big day had arrived.

As they gathered in the Priests parlor, Aznive and Mable stood in as witnesses.

An interesting custom in Armenian weddings is the "azapbashi" close to what we might refer to as the best man, and 'kavor,' or godfather in Armenian culture. The kavor is the most important figure in the wedding except for the bride and groom. In this wedding, he was AD Magarian, the groom's older brother. The Magarian's and Struel's were seated in a front row of chairs during the ceremony.

After the wedding a formal meal for family and friends supervised by the kavor, was held in the

Broadway hotel restaurant, which enhanced the prestige of the wedding couple. Dr. Magarian dressed in a black vested suit, and his bride in a loose, tubular white wedding gown with a dropped waist below knee length. They didn't go all out since the wedding took place in the parlor and not in the church. The doctor was smiling the entire time, being very proud of his new wife.

Radios were blasting throughout the hotel that Calvin Coolidge was elected President of the United States. making it the first election to be significantly influenced by radio broadcasts and a time when many Americans desired economic prosperity and peace, reflected in the "Keep cool with Collidge" campaign slogan. It was the first radio election. The radio allowed citizens across the nation to listen to political broadcasts, which was a new development that permanently changed elections.

The doctor and Pauline had plans to leave immediately after the big dinner to take the train to Niagara Falls, N.Y., which was known as the Honeymoon Capital of the World since the early 1800s, and became a popular romantic destination for newlyweds. The development of the rail lines and the

Erie Canal made the falls more accessible to a broader range of people beyond the wealthy, leading to a tourism boom. The stunning and powerful scenery of the falls provided a natural romantic and captivating backdrop for honeymooners.

A week later the couple returned to East St. Louis where they were met by AD and Gulvart Magarian. On the way to AD's home, he told them that their new house was competed and the workers were planting trees and finishing the landscaping, and the house was ready for them, except for the furniture. He turned to the doctor, and said, "Your car is filled and ready to go."

The next several days the newlyweds stayed with AD and Gulvart and their family: Aznive (25 years old and her husband Henry and their son Haig one year old), Roxie (23), Albert (9), Anahid (7) and Alphonse (5).

The next day they went to town to purchase furniture. Several days later the house was filled with new furniture and the couple were ready to move in. Before they entered, the doctor picked up his bride but barely made it across the threshold. It was quite a challenge for him since she was a head taller.

"I was hoping you wouldn't drop me," Pauline said, as they both laughed.

"I didn't know if I was going to make it," he said.

As they walked through their home. Pauline found it hard to believe that this was theirs. She never dreamed she would be blessed with such a nice home, coming from a blue-collar family and not having much education. And married to a doctor! In praying her rosary every day, she never failed to give thanks for her husband for all he had provided for her.

Part Nine

Magarian Children

CHAPTER

13

Five years later, the Magarian's had their first child, a 10 lb. baby boy. Leon Kordan Magarian, was born on August 1, 1929. He was named after his father, and given the middle name of his uncle, the one killed by the Turks in Armenia.

A year later, their second son, Robert Armanag Magarian, a 12 lb. baby boy, born on July 27, 1930. The mother gave him the name Robert (that's me) and they chose AD's name Armanag as Robert's middle name, but it was misspelled on the birth certificate, and later Robert modified it to Armen (to represent Armenia) when he was older. Five years later, their third son, Edward Oscar Magarian was born on October 3, 1935. Our mother selected her father's name, Oscar, for Edward's middle name. The doctor, who always wanted boys, was now very proud of his three sons.

My father delivered me in our home. Mom didn't make it to the hospital. I don't remember if Leon and Ed were born in the hospital or in our home.

As I was growing up in the late 30s and attending Jefferson elementary school, I learned how dedicated my father was to his profession and how he loved his patients. We didn't see him as often as we liked because of his office hours, hospital schedule, and house calls. Consequently, we went everywhere with our mother to buy our clothes, school books, church, and even to the movies.

Dr. Magarian had a busy schedule. He rose every morning around eight, had a light breakfast and went to the hospital for rounds and to see his patients. His office hours were from 11:00am – 2:00 pm, but he never left before 4:00 pm. Then he went on house calls, if there were any. He would usually arrive home around five and have his lunch. When finished he would lie down every evening for one hour then rise, have a cup of coffee and get ready to go back to his office for his 7:00 pm -10 pm evening hours.

While he was resting, mom often recorded calls from patients who needed the doctor to come to their homes. Those house calls were made after finishing his evening hours. When he finally came home around 9:30 or10:30 sometimes sooner if the evening patients were fewer and there were no house calls. He would have his late dinner and visit with mom and us. Many nights, he'd read and write.

He only had Sundays off.

In my early teens, I asked him why he had evening hours when the doctors downtown didn't, nor any others that I was aware of. He told me that many of his patients were blue-collar workers that worked in the local factories and couldn't take off work to bring in their sick family members until after work.

One morning around 7:00 am, my brother Leon and I were sitting at the kitchen table eating our Jack Armstrong Wheaties. Jack was a fictional radio star on a program that marketed Wheaties as the Breakfast of Champions. Promoting Jack as the "All-American Boy" enticed us to buy the cereal. We enjoyed listening to his radio program,

While eating our breakfast, I asked my mother where was my dad.

"He's on a Confinement Case," she said.

"What's that?" I asked.

"It's when a lady is ready to have her baby and is confined in the home," she said. "Your dad has to stay with her until the baby comes."

"Why doesn't she go to the hospital?" Leon asked

"They don't do that much these days," Mom said. "Most folks can't afford the hospital."

Leon and I remembered our parents talking about the 1929 stock market crash and the closing of the banks, and that we were living in hard times. Lots of people were out of work and many were in bread lines. Leon and I didn't quite understand all that at the time.

While we were eating breakfast this one morning, our dad drove to the back of the house in his black 1930 Model A and got out. We could see him through the back windows carrying something. When he came in, he was greeted with a kiss from mom and he put three carton of eggs on the table and got himself a cup of coffee and sat with us.

I asked, "Where did you get the eggs, Hydig" (the name for father in Armenian that we boys modified a little). We knew our dad never went shopping. Mom did it all. There were only neighborhood grocery stores, no supermarkets, and there were many street merchants peddling their fruits and vegetables, pots and pans, and the milkman delivered milk to our front steps every morning.

"My patient couldn't afford to pay me so her husband gave me these eggs," Hydig said.

"Do the eggs pay you enough for bringing their baby into the world?" Leon asked.

Hydig smiled. "It doesn't matter. These are hard times and people need our help. I hope you remember our talks about the '29 stock market crash and that there are many poor souls out of work and struggling to feed their families."

"But how are we going to eat and get our clothes?" I asked, worried that we won't have enough money.

"Boys, don't worry. We are doing fine," he said. "We

just can't waist things. You boys must learn to save."

Many of my classmates at school went barefooted during the summer to save their shoes for the fall when school started. I learned that many families suffered severe financial hardship, causing them to become very thrifty, growing vegetable gardens, and wearing patched clothing. The teenagers in the families I knew worked odd jobs to help the family put food on the table while their father was out looking for work. Unemployment was at 25%, resulting in widespread poverty, food rationing, and the loss of homes. Many teenagers often left school to help.

While we never discussed it, I sensed there were times our dad felt bad that he couldn't spend more time with us boys. Once when he was away at a medical meeting, we went to bed before he returned. During the night, I turned in my bed and something above my head moved and scared me so that I jumped out of bed and turned on the lights. There hung a Snicker candy bar tied to a string and attached to the headboard rim. One for me and one attached to Leon's bed. He woke up when I flipped on the lights and wondered what was going on.

We both laughed when we saw the candy bar dangling, knowing it was our dad who did it to tell us he loved us.

Our mother had us doing chores around the house— clean our rooms, dust, and mop the floors and clean the bathroom. She would inspect our work to make sure we did things properly. One chore I disliked the most was washing day. We had a wash machine in the basement close to a sink and a floor drain. The wash machine had a hose attached to its side, and rollers fixed at the top. We would fill the tub inside with hot water from filling several buckets at the sink. Once the tub was filled at the desired level, the clothes were added along with the soap and bleach when needed. After the cycling of the wash was done, the soapy water was removed by lowering the hose down into the floor drain. Buckets of fresh hot rinse water had to be added to the washer to remove all the soap, and then the rinse water was removed by lowering the hose again into the drain. After all the water was removed the clothes were put through the rollers at the top to squeeze out all the water; then the clothes fell into a basket on the floor. We'd then carried the basket outside to hang the clothes on several clothes lines, propping up the weight of the lines with wooden poles. Nothing smelled better than the clothes that dried in the sun and fresh air. I enjoyed their smell as we folded the clothes.

⁞•⁞

When we reached our teens, my brothers and I learned that our kitchen table where our family gathered at every meal was an expression of authority, especially the supper meal (not called dinner back then) every evening where we boys were participants. We had assignments — help mom, set the table, remove settings from the table after the meal, wash the dishes and put everything away. It's called responsibilities. We learned that this time together mattered. It was like a spiritual experience where we felt the closeness of each member of our family.

The evening meal brought us all together, and we'd sit for a couple of hours talking during and after the meal. That's where I learned our family values and what our parents expected, and what they'd tolerate from us. It was especially great when our father was with us. We'd talk about everything. How was school? What did you learn today? If anything was bothering us we'd bring it up. There were no cell phones, TVs, or computers to interrupt this sacred time together. In today's world, the kitchen table has become a place for backpacks, computers, tablets, and cell phones.

The only thing I didn't like was arguing with Leon about who was going to wash the dishes, and who was going to dry and put everything away. He only wanted to wash the dishes and left Ed and I to dry and put everything away and cover the table.

Our kitchen table also became an expression of kindness and welcome. I remember two events that occurred at our dinner table when we were teenagers, which involved our dad. This one evening, Hydig turned to mom and asked where Uncle Willy Struel and his wife were staying. They had come from Ottawa, Illinois where our mother was born, to visit grandpa Struel, his brother. Grandma Struel had two sleeping rooms upstairs that she rented out to men who worked at the brewery and went home for the weekend. We all assumed Uncle Willy and his wife were staying there.

Our mother was a little quiet at first.

"Well, are they at your folks?" he asked.

"No. They're in a motel."

"A motel?!" Hydig said, almost coming out of his chair.

"You know my mother doesn't like Uncle Willy's wife."

"Doesn't matter. They're family." He turned to Leon. Call the motel and tell them you are coming after them. They are staying here."

As it turned out, we had a great time together.

Another event that happened at our dinner table, which demonstrated my dad's kindness and thoughtfulness occurred when this black man (I forget his name) that did handy work around the grounds of our home came to the door and Leon showed him to our kitchen. He stood by the table and told Hydig that he had finished and he was leaving and would return the next day. My dad told him to sit at the table next to him and have dinner with us. He told me to get a plate and setting for the man. Our handyman hesitated and said he wasn't hungry. My dad insisted that he sit and at least have some dessert and coffee. He removed his cap and sat in the chair but didn't pull it up to the table. Hydig motioned for him to move in more to the table. He did, but he wouldn't eat.

"Then you must have a piece of my wife's delicious pie and some coffee, Hydig said, as mom placed a slice of cherry pie in front of him and filled his cup with coffee. He nodded rather awkwardly. "Thank you."

We all tried to make him feel comfortable asking about his family. He finally seemed at ease and just smiled. Mom made a plate of food for him to take home.

Part Ten

World War II

14

The decade of the thirties was about to end and a grand innovation was about to take place –the introduction of the dial telephone –on January first, 1940. Before the new decade arrived, we were accustomed to interacting with the telephone operator to place our calls. We'd lift the receiver and say, "Operator, please ring . . ." whatever number we were calling. Our home phone number was "East 212."

Ninety-nine percent of the operators were females and at times a good friend of the family, Virgina Moomjian, would see our number on her board and when she heard my voice, she'd say, "Bobby, is that you?"

I'd respond, "Hi, Virginia. How are you and your mom doing?" Her mother was a very close friend of my mother's, who lived on Natalie Avenue, the street behind us. If the operator rang the number you asked for, and it was busy, she'd tell you so, and that you should try again later. They were always very pleasant and helpful. As a reminder: my mother was a telephone operator before marrying my dad.

We had received our new home dial phones and played with them like a new toy. We couldn't wait until the day and time came when we could dial the new numbers that were published. Of course, we dialed our relatives and everyone we knew. We had fun getting used to the new system. It took a couple of days before my brothers and I got tired of it.

We lived just a block from our uncle AD's home where I would spend much of my free time, sitting in the screened-in porch with my aunt, grandma, and my cousins. I learned a lot about the Armenian culture and enjoyed some of the Middle Eastern fruit snacks—fruits, figs and dates. Sometimes they'd send me across the street to Parkway Inn for soft drinks. Parkway Inn was a cozy restaurant with a huge parking lot, which became a hangout for high school students on the weekends.

My grandmother couldn't speak English but she could say "7-UP," her favorite drink. I enjoyed being with her even though we couldn't carry on a conversation. There was something about her kindness and warmth that attracted me to her. She used to sit in her rocker and pray her black beads, which always remined me that my grandfather, her husband, was an Armenian Orthodox priest. Just being in her company made me feel something spiritual. This time she looked at me and said, "Bobby, Tsitik (pronounced (sock-es, which affectionately means little bird) 7-up." She got up and I followed her slowly upstairs to her room. She was small, short and in her nineties. In her room she opened the lower drawer of her chifforobe and pulled out her purse. Once she opened it, I pulled out a $20 bill to tease her, and she grabbed it back, shook her head and spoke. "No, no, honey," and gave me a five-dollar bill. She couldn't speak English but like all Armenians, she knew her money. After I got back from Parkway Inn with the 7-up we sat and enjoyed our sodas as she just smiled at me.

Mission accomplished. This was one of my rare occasions when I spent time with my lovely grandmother.

Nearly every Sunday our father and mother and we three boys joined our uncle's family for a big dinner meal (back then dinner was the noon meal) that the ladies spent a lot of time preparing. The meal consisted mainly of Armenian dishes, lots of fruit, and pastry. It was oh, so good! We all sat at the dining room table in the dining area that opened a few feet from the large living room. There were our five, uncle AD, auntie Gulvart, cousin Aznive, her husband Henry Apoian, and their son, Haig, and cousins Albert and Alphonse (who had the nickname "Bus"). You can imagine all the happy times we had talking over one another and all the laughter.

This Sunday, December 7th, 1941, we all were together again having our dinner. When we finished, the men went into the living room. My uncle turned on the radio and after about fifteen minutes of listening to the music, it was interrupted with a special announcement from the White House. My uncle called out to the women. "Come, I think the President is going to speak."

They came and stood behind their husband's chairs.

This was an official announcement coming from The White House around 1:00 p.m. EST. The man who spoke had a serious tone in his voice. He confirmed that Japanese forces had bombed Pearl Harbor and other locations in the Pacific, and we were told that the president would appear before Congress on Monday, December 8, 1941 to ask Congress to declare war on the Empire of Japan,

Everyone in the room became quiet. Shock filled their faces. Aznive looked at her son, Haig, who was 18, and my uncle and aunt looked at their sons, Albert and Bus, who were in their 20s. They certainly would be of age to be drafted into the military.

I distinctly remember asking: "Does that mean Haig, Albert, and Bus will be going to war?" No one answered. I looked around the room at the faces filled with fear. Finally my dad said, "We'll have to wait and see."

President Roosevelt did appear before Congress the next day on December 8, 1941 and gave his famous "Day of Infamy" speech addressing the December 7 surprise attack on Pearl Harbor by Japan. He labeled the date as one that will live in infamy, declaring the attack "dastardly" and unprovoked and immediately asked Congress to declare a state of war.

What surprised me days later were the millions of young and older men volunteering for the armed forces, not waiting for letters from their draft boards. All the newspapers and magazines had many pictures of young men standing in line smiling while waiting to register for the draft. Anyone 18 and older were ordered to immediately go to their designated locations to register. I was 11, too young.

The culture of our nation began to change. Sixteen million men went to WWII, while the women left their homes to became our heroes, going into the manufacturing roles to make, ships, airplanes, tanks, and ammunition. The ladies were given the name of "Rosie the Riveter," a portrait posted all over, which represented the workers dressed in working jeans, a red and white polka dot bandana, and work boots. Rosie was mostly depicted as standing on the wing of an airplane putting in rivets.

The children of the workers were cared for through a combination of federal, private, and community networks, neighbors, relatives, and even rotating care systems among working mothers became involved. There was a massive rationing of gasoline, food, clothing, and significant social changes. To manage shortages, the government rationed meat, sugar, butter, tires and gasoline, and citizens used coupons, and for many gasoline was limited to 4 gallons per week.

The economy shifted to full-time war production with factories operating 24/7.

I remember many families planted "victory gardens" (20 million gardens producing 45% of US vegetables by 1945) and participated in scrap metal and rubber drives. We collected all the silver wrappings around cigarette packs and turned in balls of silver to the government agencies.

We relied heavily on radio for news, while movie theatres showed news reels about the war. But we went to the movies to escape from the fear of all we read.

I can't help but think about the sacrifices everyone made at that time, men who had families went to war for four years before returning home. Such a sacrifice for their wives. too. Just imagine, a man having two children, ages 1 and 2 years old, and when he returned after four years his children would be 5 and 6 years of age. They wouldn't know daddy, except from the pictures their mother showed them to keep his memory alive. I was in Korea for 15 months and thank God it wasn't 4 years. I can relate to the sacrifices those men and women endured, being separated from each other for 4 years. The "Greatest Generation."

Part Eleven

Peacetime – Change in the Culture of Medicine

15

During the war effort, medical scientists searched for an anti-infective agent to treat battle wounds. Fortunately, penicillin was discovered and the penicillin mold cultures were first grown in thousands of milk bottles, bed pans, and huge milk churns. Massive amounts were needed for the military and the industrial deep-tank fermentation processes finally took over to scale up the badly needed production of the antibiotic.

In March 1942, penicillin was tried on the first civilian patient in the U.S. By 1945, massive amounts were now in production. Penicillin became widely used to treat allied forces during the D-Day invasion in 1945 on the beaches of Normandy, France. It proved highly effective in treating wound infections, pneumonia, and other bacterial diseases in the mid-forties.

The drug became widely available to the public later in 1946, and was called the "Miracle Drug."

Before 1945, my father ordered an early batch of penicillin that came in multidose vials. Each vial was filled with a light brown liquid, which was stored in the fridge. Multidose meant that my dad had to withdraw a single dose from the bottle into a syringe multiple times to treat his patients. It was used in his office primarily for syphilis and gonorrhea. Before penicillin, I was aware that the doctors only had sulfa and Salvarsan (arsphenamine) or called "compound 606," which was the first effective modern antibiotic agent introduced in 1910 by Paul Ehrlich to treat syphilis. As the first "magic bullet" this arsenic -based drug targeted specific pathogens and was the primary treatment for syphilis until being replaced by penicillin in the 1940s. Salvarsan was notoriously unstable, toxic, and required careful intravenous administration. Adverse effects included extreme pain at the injection site—lasting days—rashes, liver damage, fever, vomiting, diarrhea, and risks of arsenic poisoning. Despite toxicity, tens of thousands of doses were administered by 1910.

All that the doctors had in the forties to assist in their practice were — X-ray, blood work, and urine analysis — no CT scan, MRI, or PET scan. There was far less technology with greater reliance on doctor-patient relationships. Doctors often worked long hours, a stark difference from modern medicine.

I went to my dad's office on some weekends and evenings, to straighten up and alphabetize his medicine closet, which was filled with meds he ordered along with those left by professional drug reps. This middle room separated two large examining rooms. My dad's desk was in this middle room where the patients would sit while he wrote their prescriptions, and explained more about his diagnosis, and what he wanted them to do. There were times he'd ask me to get sheets out of the drawers in the large cabinet against the wall that contained instructions and/or dietary restrictions to give to the patients.

He taught me the few lab tests that we performed in the little lab, which was also in this middle room, and allowed me to be in the examination room with him with his male patients that agreed to allow me to be in the room to observe even though I was only 15 years old. My dad told them I was in training as a young man for medical school. Most were pleased, and many asked me, "Are you going to be as good as your dad?"

"I hope so," I said, glancing at my dad, who smiled.

When I turned 17, I spent more time at the office performing certain tasks, such as, analyzing urine samples collected from the patients, and took their vital signs to record in their notebooks. I wore a white jacket to look professional, and my dad allowed me to assist him with his female patients when he didn't have to examine their private areas. If that were determined, I would leave the room and the nurse would assist him. I was allowed to be with the male patients during their examination and treatment processes.

The new batches of multidose vials of penicillin we now received were more purified and had a light ivory color. I was taught how to administer the shots in men's hips, and got pretty good at it.

Around 1947, we were purchasing sterile disposable

syringes of penicillin containing different doses — 100,000 units and 200, 000 units that didn't have to be refrigerated. My dad would tell me what dosage to administer to the man in the examining room when we came out. It was either for gonorrhea or syphilis. I'd pull out the drawer and get the disposable unit and go in and ask the patient to drop his pants so I could administer the shot in his hip. It felt good helping someone.

Out in the waiting room, the nurse would ask who was next to see the doctor. It was first-come-first-serve. No appointments were ever scheduled.

I remember well this one case — a heavy-set black lady that the nurse brought into the front examining room. She let me take the patient's vitals and collect a urine sample from her to test for sugar in our little lab. I would enter all the data in her notebook that the nurse put on the side table close to the door and next to the chair the patient sat in.

This patient, Mattie James, in her fifties, had high blood pressure and was diabetic. After examining her urine, I found sugar in the test tube. I was thinking: *my dad isn't going to like this.* When he came into the room, he greeted Ms. James (I don't remember her actual name; I couldn't give it if I did). My dad was always very friendly and kind towards his patients, which impressed me. He tapped Ms. James on the shoulder and said, "How are you today, Mattie?"

"Oh, doctor, I could be better."

He stood next to her looking over her data in the book on the table next to her chair and turned back to her and said, "Have you been a good girl following the diet I gave you, and taking your insulin?" Of course, he knew she hadn't.

Mattie, bowed her head and shook it a little and said, "Dr. Magarian," then got quiet for a few seconds, "It was Thanksgiving and I had to have that extra piece of Pumpkin Pie."

"Are you sure you didn't have more?"

She smiled looking down at the floor, "I plan to do better, doctor."

He tapped her on the shoulder, again, then said," Mattie, tell me something."

"Yes, doctor."

"How long do you want to live?"

She quickly turned to him with and expression of fear and surprise. "Well, doctor, I want to live as long as I can."

"You will if you do as I say, but I can't guarantee anything if you don't follow my instructions."

"Oh, doctor, I promise I'll do whatever you say from now on."

"Good. I want you to stay on the diet we gave you, take your insulin, and don't skip any doses, and I want you to lose 5 pounds in the next two weeks." He paused. "Can you do that for me?"

"Yes, doctor. I promise."

"Good. That's what I like to hear," he said patting her on the shoulder, again. "Then you'll be fine, Mattie."

"Thank you, doctor," she said, smiling. As she stood to leave, I thought she was about to hug him.

My dad took me aside and said, "There are a couple of practices in medicine that must be followed in making an accurate diagnosis. One, you must listen to the patient. They will give you a lot of information as they describe their symptoms. That helps tremendously. Also, the doctor must always show compassion for his patients. It makes them feel relaxed and allows them to open-up. Showing that you care is half of the healing process and makes for a good bedside manner."

One afternoon while I was with my dad he received a call from Barnes Hospital in St. Louis, an institution equivalent to Mayo Clinic. I was sitting in the chair next to his desk when he took the call. The doctor in charge told my dad that they had examined his female patient, and they felt that they had come up with a different diagnosis. My dad told him that was fine, all he wanted was for them to treat her. I realized my dad wasn't affected by the call, he was more concerned about doing what was needed for his patient. Interestingly, two days later, I happened to be in the office again when Barnes called. They said they had finished all their testing and had determined his diagnosis was correct, and they wanted him to know that and they were proceeding with her treatment, and would have her contact him for a follow up appointment when she was released. My dad thanked them and hung up.

I told him how pleased I was for him. He told me the only thing that matters is what's best for the patient.

I was proud of my dad!

I remember another case where we had dressed the whole right arm of a lady patient who had received very bad burns. My father told me to remove the dressing from her arm so she could be treated while he was treating another patient in the other room. I began removing the bandage from the top of her shoulder, wetting the dressing as I cut the bandage away. As I pulled on the bandage, inch-by-inch, she jumped and cried out every time I pulled it down. I did my best to keep her from feeling any pain, but she still yelled. I got a third of the way down with some of the bandage hanging down under her arm. My dad came into the room to get something, and as he entered, he quickly grabbed the hanging bandage and pulled it forward in one swift motion, pulling it completely off. She jumped up in her seat and let out one big yell. He said as he went out, "You only had to feel the pain once." She looked at me as she sat down. "He's right," she said. "Better than what you were doing."

I thought, *Okay, dear lady. Next time I'll do the same when you come in.*

Another event that sticks with me was one evening in the office when we were finishing up and about to close the office and go home, I went out to the waiting room to arrange the chairs and stack the magazines and about to lock the door when this black man entered, drunk and bleeding from the neck. He looked at me with bloodshot eyes and with slurring words, "Is the doc here?"

I wasn't happy to see him. I wanted to go home, it was about 9:45 pm.

"What happened to you," I asked, as I grabbed him to keep him from falling.

It took him a few seconds to answer. "My sister cut me."

"Let's go to the back," I said holding him so he wouldn't fall. "Why did she cut you?" I asked.

"We got into a fight."

He stumbled again. I stabilized him and then led him into the back examining room, and got him up on the examining table, and I told him to lie back. I then went to get Hydig, who was about to take off his white jacket.

"I got this drunk on the table. He's bleeding from his neck. Said his sister cut him."

"Let's take a look," he said.

When we entered the room, the man was groaning.

"What's your name? Hydig asked as he unbuttoned the man's shirt.

"Abraham," he finally said as I helped pull his shirt open to put a sterile towel under his neck while my dad gloved up to examine the wound. I got the sutures, forceps, sanitizer, and ethyl chloride spray to lessen the pain, and put them on the side tray.

"The wound isn't too deep," Hydig said.

I cleaned the wound and sprayed a little ethyl chloride on it as Hyding sutured it closed. When he had finished, Hydig pulled off his gloves, threw them into the special container, and told me to put on the dressing, and he went into the middle room. When done, I asked the man how he was doing.

"Good. The doc is good."

"That he is," I said, and helped him off the table. He stood for a few seconds and seemed much better. He went into the middle room while I cleaned up.

When I came out, Hydig was putting on his coat.

I asked, "Where did the man go? I didn't get his full name or address. Do you know him?"

"Never saw him before."

I hurried into the waiting room and opened the door and he was gone.

I hurried back. "He's gone."

"Forget it."

I realized my dad didn't care about the money. He helped a man in need, and that was good enough for him.

ↄ•Ↄ

After the war ended in 1945, postwar medicine began to change. Our family was shocked the day our dad came home and told us that during the hospital staff meeting the doctors voted to no longer make house calls. We were to tell call-ins to take the patients to the ER. I knew in my heart it was the doctors who came home from the war that pushed for no house calls. My dad said one doctor in the meeting said, "The doctor making the house call can't take an x-ray machine along with him." I didn't find that amusing. If an x-ray were needed, then the patient would go to the hospital.

I thought, *my dad did okay. Rarely did he have to send a patient to the hospital.*

It wasn't long after that all the doctors began taking an additional weekday off besides Sunday. The culture of medicine was about to change.

Part Twelve

Turning Point in the Practice of Medicine

CHAPTER
16

The 1950s are considered the turning point in the history of medicine.

This started with the discovery of penicillin in the forties, which led to the creation of generations of powerful antibiotics. The most troublesome illness of that time was polio, infantile paralysis, until Jonas Salk developed an effective vaccine. Scarlet fever, pneumonia, smallpox were also troubling. Most of the population received the smallpox vaccine that left a scar on the arm. During that period, physicians had the autonomy to deliver highly personal health care, because federally mandated regulations were few and constraints from insurance companies were almost nonexistent, and the doctors had the authority to deliver highly personal health care. Most physician were in private practice.

They often prescribed the most popular drugs in the 50s that were amphetamines for housewives that wanted to have a boost of energy and to lose weight, and barbiturates were used to treat anxiety and insomnia. Both had a high tendency for abuse.

Modern medicine differs drastically from the 50s, shifting from a paternalistic house-call model to a highly technological specialized and data-driven industry. Key changes include advanced imaging (MRI, CT, Pet Scan) molecular diagnostic, targeted therapies, minimal invasive surgeries, and the rise of Evidence-based Medicine (EBM).

EBM is a systematic approach to clinical care that integrates the best available research evidence with clinical expertise and patient values to make informed healthcare decisions.

Todays practice of medicine is a focus on chronic diseases, personalized medicine, surgical complex procedures and greater understanding of genetic and complex conditions. In the 1940s doctors often worked unpaid in hospitals as a condition of staff privileges. Early beginnings of group practice came after wartime experiences.

Doctors have increasingly moved into group practices affiliated with hospitals and medical institutions to combat financial, administrative, and clinical pressures of running a private practice. The percentage of doctors in private practice dropped from 60% in 2012 to 47% in 2022, while hospitals employed positions increased.

The reasons the doctors made this switch is: financial stability, reduced risk with hospitals that offered a steady salary compared to the declining income from private practice, rising costs from malpractice insurance -fear of being sued-overhead, and administrative costs, like electronic health records. Group practices and hospital affiliations allow doctors a greater leverage to negotiate higher payment rates with insurance companies, which is a major factor for 80% of doctors selling their practices.

₧•₨

Still, the practice of medicine faces many challenges, characterized by a shift from patient-oriented care to a system dominated by administrative technology and financial pressures. Key down sides include high rates of clinical burnout, the erosion of the physician-patient relationship, and looking ahead to 2026 as a worsening affordability crisis for patients.

Here are summarized primary concerns to the practice of medicine in the current scene.

1. Physicians burden and burnout. They spend much more time on electronic health records (EHRs) and desk work than on direct patient care, often a couple of hours of desk work for every hour of face time.

2. Burnout Epidemic. Over 45% of our physicians report symptoms of burnout in 2024, driven by excessive workloads, and the lack of control and relentless administrative tasks.

3. A critical shortage of nurses and physicians is expected to worsen with projections of up to 3-4 million fewer healthcare workers than needed this year due to an aging workforce, high turnover and fewer professionals entering the field.

4. The erosion of patient- doctor relationships.

Technology is a barrier while EHR offer efficiency, they often act as a barrier between doctor and patient, reducing in-person connections.

5. The need for efficiency and high-volume billing has significantly cut into the time available for listening to and examining patients, being replaced by high-tech impersonal care, which has led to the patient's trust in the medical system to decline because care feels hurried or impersonal.

6. Rising costs and low reimbursements, while operational costs, including labor and supplies, are soaring, Medicare and insurance reimbursements are not keeping up with inflation. As high deductible plans become the norm, patents are increasingly postponing or skipping necessary care due to cost.

7. Corporate medicine has caused independent practices to disappear with most being acquired by hospital s or private equity, which can depersonalize care and increase costs.

8. Physicians spend hours weekly fighting insurance companies to get treatment approval for patients.

9. The clinical skills are in danger of being lost. The

over-reliance on testing — the ease of ordering imaging (CT, MRI) and lab tests has led to a decline in physical exam skills and bedside diagnosis.

10. Modern medicine often focuses on fixing a lab value rather than treating the whole patient.

11. Physicians often experience moral injury when they are unable to provide the care they believe is right due to administrative or financial constraints.

12. Physicians fear of lawsuits from lawyers for misdiagnosis.

In conclusion, the above analysis reveals that these factors have created a challenging environment, particularly in primary care, where many practitioners are considering leaving the field due to the relentless pressures.

(Notice: The above AI overview content has been reviewed, verified and edited by the author)

During his decades my dad embraced the advances in technology and pharmaceuticals that gave him greater insight into the illnesses plaguing his patients and better means to treat them, he was still bothered with the shift to increasingly corporatized medicine (transforming doctors into independent profit-oriented business-like corporations, or bringing them under corporate control) where there was the erosion of the doctor-patient relationship. Despite everything, he always remained steadfast in his convictions—above all, a doctor must listen to his patients and show compassion for their struggles—convictions that my dad passed on as his legacy.

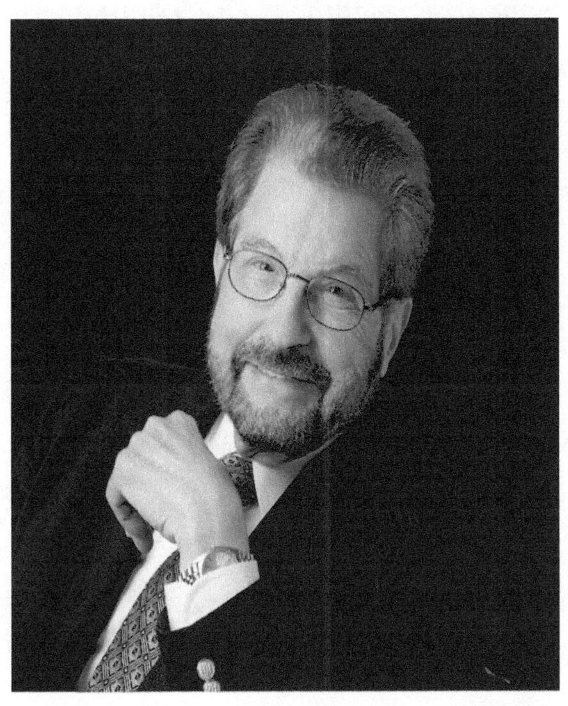

ROBERT MAGARIAN, B.A., BSPh, Ph.D., is professor emeritus of medicinal chemistry and pharmaceutics. He has been writing fiction since his retirement and has created several fictional characters in medical and detective thrillers. The two most popular characters are Detectives Cowboy Noah McGraw and Holly Roark of the Atlanta PD.

Magarian is the author of five thriller novels, *The Watchman, Seventy-Two Hours, You'll Never See Me*

Again, A Crime to Remember, The Tongue Collector, and *Forever Young*.

In addition to his fiction, Magarian is the author of his latest nonfiction book: *Amazing Love, It Can Be, a Memoir*. He has also written two essays: *Follow Your Dream*, and *A Journey into Faith*. He lives with his family in Norman, Oklahoma.

www.ingramcontent.com/pod-product-compliance
Lightning Source LLC
Chambersburg PA
CBHW021221130726
47988CB00002B/761